Gout,
- and how I tamed it.

By C. E. Cox

Spring 2024

Table of Contents

Introduction

This book is a personal record of my journey and experiences over many years, and how I eventually came to tame gout.

I would like to say I have beaten it, but that isn't true as I still get flare-ups.

A fellow sufferer used to say he didn't have gout because he took pills for it. I argued that if he stopped taking the pills then it world return, hence he still had gout.

By taming gout, I mean that I do not have to take any pills, and I can avoid serious attacks by using the methods described here.

Most people with gout will find some of their experiences match and others not. We are all different and often some of the triggers foods for a gout attack vary considerably, as do the cures.

It is an extremely painful condition that renders you unable to walk, or move far, and

so knowing how to avoid attacks can
prevent lots of misery, and time off work.

Disclaimer

I offer this information solely on the basis of
my personal experiences and as a layman,
and I cannot be considered any sort of
medical expert. You must consult a doctor if
you are suffering from gout, as they can
prescribe beneficial medication.

The Early years

The Large Big Toe

I was in my late 40's when I found my right big toe was very large and very painful, so eventually I made an appointment with the GP, and was sent me for an X-ray which showed nothing, and had no idea what was wrong other than calling it a Bunion.

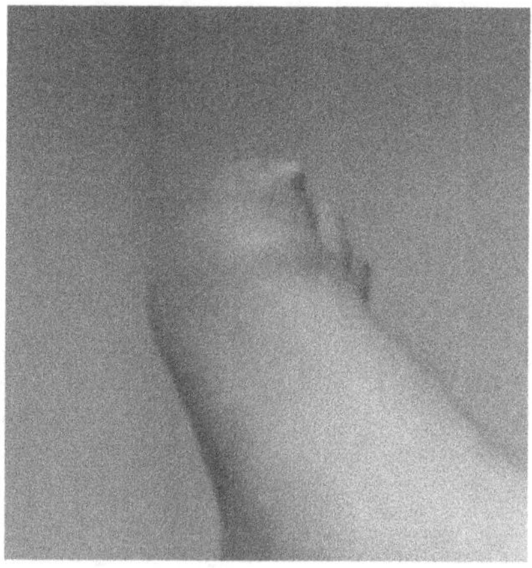

I dreaded getting new shoes as the right shoe took ages to break in and the leather expand enough around the toe to make them comfortable.

In hindsight it seems to me to that it was a pre-cursor to gout, because later I was affected in the same place by gout, and so believe it is all part of the same problem.

I was drinking beer and some ales at the time with wine at meals but rarely touched sprits, and the problem seemed to diminish for a while.

Knobbly hands

Lets be honest, you will probably not suffer with gout if you are not a regular drinker.

It is hard to quantify how much is too much, but drinking every day with a few binge sessions over say 10 years is going to put you in the frame.

In the 2000s I started to notice my hands
were somewhat deformed, with lumps and
bumps near the joints.

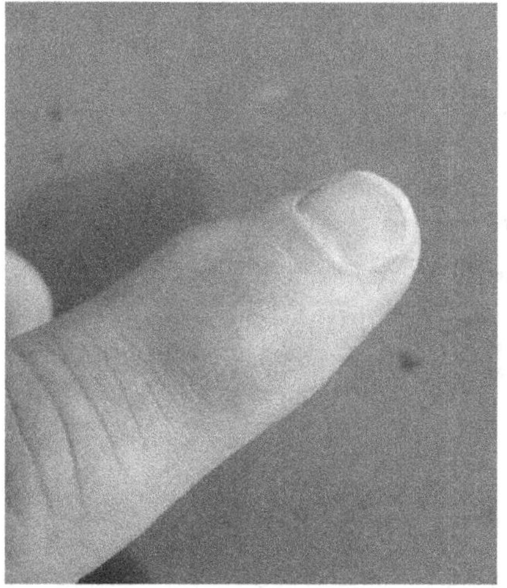

These could become painful and I was
mystified as to the cause, Googling revealed
a possible cause which is Heberden's nodes

or Bouchard's nodes depending on which joints are affected.

They're caused by the growth of bony spurs called osteophyte.

Osteoarthritis can affect anyone at any age, but it's more common in women over the age of 50.

My mother suffered from it, but I took the excellent supplement chondroitin, and glucosamine which rebuilds cartilage and that helped, but it didn't stop the attacks.

Eventually I realised this was just another form of gout, which after a year of treatment with Allopurinol reduced these growths considerably.

Getting Serious

Massive foot and knee swelling

In the late 2000's my drinking increased due to marital problems which meant I was usually in the pub 6-10pm and then getting up at 7am to head off to work.

Dark Navy Rum was a favourite "one for the road" and I started to experience attacks in my feet, knees, ankles, and thumbs.

These progressively got worse in pain, duration and frequency. Eventually I went to the doctor who prescribed Allopurinol which did reduce the frequency of attacks.

During lockdown I had a bad attack and was unable to walk, but being out of work at the time, it was no major issue.

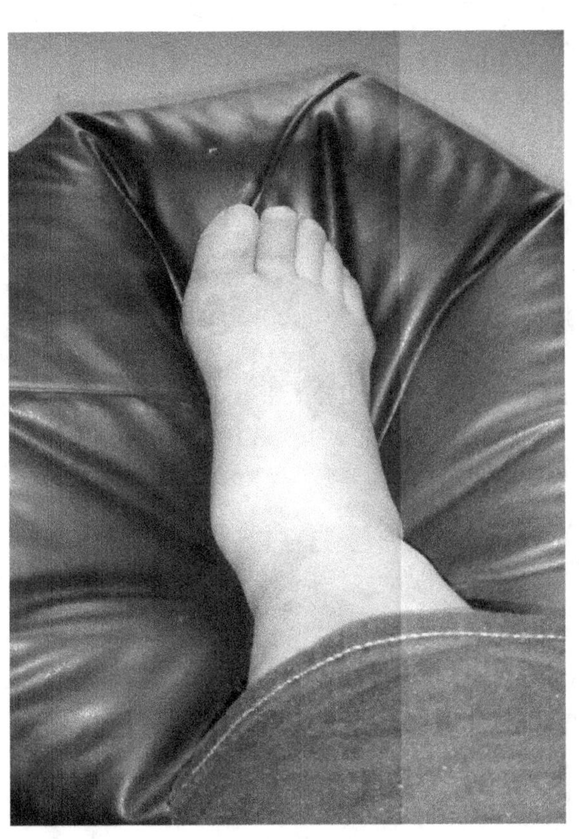

Getting the medication however was, eventually a friend picked them up for me which included Colchicine, and as they started to take effect I started to do some google research in my ample free time.

Since that time I always ensure I have a least six tables of Colchicine in case of an attack, as it can take days to get any further medication, and it is best taken as early as possible.

What is going wrong

So what is gout?

Gout is a form of arthritis caused by uric acid crystals that form in and around joints.

Uric acid is a normal part of body waste created when chemicals called purines are broken down by your kidneys.

Many foods and drinks are high in purines, some of which I have listed under Trigger Foods.

The body usually excretes this acid through waste, but if the kidneys are over-loaded it can collect in the blood.

High levels of uric acid in the blood can form crystals in the joints, and this is the cause of gout.

Drinking lots of water can help flush out uric acid and so 1 litre a day would be a good basis of treatment.

The Engine

Basically your liver and kidneys are like any engine, the harder you work it the less efficient it becomes.

The capacity to process alcohol and protein diminishes with age, as your bodies' ability to do the work decreases with use.

However this is only part of the problem. Trappers in Alaska often died within 6 weeks of leaving town. Researchers eventually realised that the problem was that they were living solely off rabbit. Worse still, they tended to spit-roast the rabbit, which meant the lean meat was devoid of any fat.

People who have been rescued after crashing in the mountains or being stranded in the Artic ice, reportedly would drink oil straight from the bottle, they craved it so much. Human flesh is also very lean.

The crucial point is that your body needs **animal** fat to process meat protein, and alcohol, and a lot of the bad press about animal fat is simply not true, see ref 1.

It is not a coincidence that a full English breakfast is the standard hangover cure for many.

Lean Meat

Game has always been associated with gout, and anyone who has eaten pheasant, rabbit, and venison can attest to how lean it is. The media may have you believe that animal fat is bad for you as it increases cholesterol, but research has not proven this, in fact eating animal fats in one study reduced cholesterol, See ref 2.

One related experience I had was when I woke up in the morning with a bad attack, and thought back to my previous meal - which was a carvery lunch where I had eaten roast beef.

This is a fairly lean meat, but the problem was compounded by the fact that the gravy was made from a packet and not the juice and oils from the pan.

Since then, I always make gravy from the animal fats and juices left in the roasting pan.

I stick to eating venison and other game meats as burgers (which have fat), or make a stew with say pheasant and chicken.

Vegetable Oil - The big Lie

As a species we have evolved over thousands of years to live on a diet of meat, fish, and fruit. Only in the last 14K years have grains become an important part of our diet, and even so evolution is slow and many people are still wheat intolerant.

Seeds have generally never been a part of our diet, some are usually consumed as part of a fruit, but these are not broken down, but excreted whole to germinate.

There is mounting evidence that the prevailing increase in "Western Illnesses" such as heart disease, obesity and diabetes etc, are directly related to the amount of seed oil in our diet, see ref 3.

99% of packaged\processed foods contain vegetable oil, even dried fruit is covered in it, and I have only found 1 packaged product without it –some brands of shortbread biscuits.

Seed oil has the wrong sort of Omega oils that our bodies cannot easily process, and generally just store the oils as fatty tissue.

Trans oils are even worse and should be avoided at all cost.

It is worth noting that the healthy Mediterranean diet is focused on Olive oil. Oils from fruits such as olives and avocados are far better for us, and if you need hot oils, then you should use goose fat or lard.

All this seed oil adds to the burden placed on the liver and kidneys which struggle to process it, for gout suffers it is best avoided.

The Good

Gout Buster foods

There are many pages on the internet and many books devoted to anti-inflammatory foods, but to summarise here are the main ones, with the those that can also reduce uric acid:

	Anti-inflammatory	Uric acid reducer
Turmeric	Yes	
Black Cherries	Yes	Yes
Dry Cider Vinegar	Yes	
Coffee		Yes
Skimmed Milk	Yes	Yes
Water		Yes
Vitamin C		Yes
Avocado		Yes
Olive oil	Yes	
Greens	Yes	

Oily Fish	Yes	

The Bad

Trigger foods

These can vary from person to person, and so they are things to watch out for, and this is where a journal can come in handy.

I found a fellow sufferer who also loved Marmite, and had to suggest sadly it was a trigger for me and probably him as well.

Another chap seems to be averse to the Nightshade foods which I seem fine with.

It is useful to keep a journal of what you eat before the gout attack, and details of the location and length of time to recover. There is a page at the end of the book are reserved for this purpose.

Yeasty

- Marmite
- Beer

Purine Rich Foods

- Pea Shoots (raw)
- Petit Pois
- Liver and kidneys
- Turkey
- Oily Fish
- Asparagus

Nightshade foods

- Chilli
- Tomatoes (raw)
- Peppers (raw)
- Aubergine

Fructose corn syrup and Sugary Drinks

- Diet Drinks
- Baked Goods

- Fast Foods
- Some Cereals
- Honey

Shellfish

- Various

The ugly

Although all alcohol is bad for gout, if not the main cause, the stronger it is the more work the body has to perform to break down the alcohol.

High alcohol content drinks

- Port
- Spirits
- Beer over 5%
- Some herbal Tonics

Medication

These are the medicines I have used of the
last 5 years.

	Anti-inflammatory	Uric acid reducer	Comments
Allopurinol	Yes	Yes	It reduced the lumps in my hands, but after a year it seemed to be causing regular attacks.
Colchicine	Yes	Yes	Use as a last resort, but clears gout in 3 days. Avoid Grapefruit
Ibuprofin	Yes		Works well
Nabproxin	Yes		Works very well

Living with the devil

The twinge and how to deal with it

I may go many weeks with no symptoms at all, and then wake up to find a part of my hand or knee has a sore lump.

It is important to act quickly, so that morning I will take 1 Ibuprofen and 1 Turmeric tablet.

This usually nips the attack in the bud. Drinking cherry juice will help as will lots of water.

If you can add in some of the gout remedies above all the better.

For those who can take Naproxen, it is much more effective than Ibuprofen, and works more quickly. It is the best first line of defence, and in most cases will cure the twinge. If you can get it prescribed keep a stock handy.

Unfortunately, it is not prescribed to me due to another medication I am on.

Start of a serious attack, serious medicine

If the attack progress the following morning to become a swollen knee or ankle for example,

the next step for me is to take two 500 microgram Colchicine tablets.

I then follow this with 1 in the evening a 1 in the morning for 2 days or so until it clears.

This drug can kill you so you must follow the prescription advise on the packet, and avoid grapefruit.

Thankfully this regimen has worked for me
for over three years now, - but I always
ensure I have at least six Colchicine tablets
available.

Summary

If you have purchased and read this book you will not need me to remind you how painful gout is, and how debilitating it can be.

Avoiding serious attacks therefore greatly improves your levels of health and happiness.

Managing your diet is the best way to help your body stay healthy, so it is important to avoid processed foods, packet foods, vegetable oils, and sweet drinks.

However, reducing your alcohol consumption will have the biggest positive impact on gout avoidance. This can mean cutting it out completely, or drinking only low alcohol drinks.

I trust that you will then also have tamed gout, and no longer need medication.

References

Ref 1. 9 Myths About Dietary Fat and Cholesterol. https://www.healthline.com/nutrition/fat-and-cholesterol

Ref 2. Reducing the serum cholesterol level with a diet high in animal fat.

https://pubmed.ncbi.nlm.nih.gov/3336803/

Ref 3. Omega-6 Apocalypse: 'Vegetable Oils' and Western Diseases by Dr Chris Knobbe. https://www.youtube.com/watch?v=sGxc2nbV5ac

Journal

The point of keeping a journal is to build up an picture of what you have consumed prior to any signs of gout to enable you to spot which food or drink may be a trigger.

Date	Food & Drink
Date	**Symptom**

Date	Food & Drink
Date	**Symptom**

Date	Food & Drink

Date	Symptom

Date	Food & Drink
Date	Symptom

Date	Food & Drink

Date	Symptom

Date	Food & Drink

Date	Symptom

Date	Food & Drink
Date	**Symptom**

Date	Food & Drink

Date	Symptom